ESOPHAGITIS DIET COOKBOOK:

FOR NEWLY DIAGNOSED

Complete Beginner Procedures On Food

Recipes, Guided Meal Plans, And Healthy

Lifestyle Tips To Manage, Strive, And Live

Well With Esophagitis

DR. EMMY BROOKS

ABOUT THIS BOOK

In the realm of health and wellness, understanding the intricacies of a condition like Esophagitis is paramount, and that's precisely where the "Esophagitis Diet Cookbook" shines. This book serves as a guiding light, illuminating the path toward relief and comfort through a specialized diet. At its core, it seeks to demystify Esophagitis, unraveling its complexities, from its causes to its symptoms, and empowering individuals with knowledge to better navigate their journey towards wellness.

One of the key revelations within these pages is the pivotal role diet plays in managing Esophagitis. Here, readers discover the profound impact of their food choices and the importance of crafting a customized diet plan tailored to their unique needs. By recognizing trigger foods and embracing Esophagitis-friendly ingredients, individuals can lay a solid foundation for their dietary journey, paving the way for relief and comfort.

Stocking the kitchen becomes an art form with the guidance provided in this book. From essential ingredients for an Esophagitis-friendly diet to savvy grocery shopping tips, readers are equipped with the tools needed to transform their kitchen into a sanctuary of healing. Practical meal planning takes center stage, offering a weekly meal planner guide that balances both nutrients and flavor, ensuring every bite is not only nourishing but also deliciously satisfying.

Cooking becomes a joyous exploration of gentle techniques and non-aggravating recipes. Through the lens of Esophagitis-friendly cooking methods, readers discover a world where flavor and comfort coexist harmoniously. From nutrient-rich breakfasts to satisfying lunches and soothing dinners, every meal is crafted with care to provide relief and nourishment, offering respite from discomfort and heartburn.

Beyond the kitchen, this book extends its reach, guiding readers through the intricacies of navigating restaurants and embracing lifestyle changes for long-term relief. With strategies for stress reduction, incorporating exercise, and celebrating successes along the journey, it becomes more than just a cookbook—it becomes a roadmap to a life of vitality and wellness, where Esophagitis no longer holds sway over one's well-being.

DISCLAIMER:

This book's content is solely intended for general informative purposes. About the availability, applicability, correctness, completeness, and trustworthiness of the data or recipes in this book, the author provides no guarantees of any sort, either stated or implied. You bear full responsibility for any reliance you may have on such material.

The advice, diagnosis, or treatment provided by a qualified medical expert is not to be replaced by this cookbook. When in doubt about a medical problem, never hesitate to consult your doctor or another trained healthcare professional. Never ignore medical advice from professionals or put off getting it because of something you've read in this book.

At the time of publishing, the author of this book has taken reasonable steps to guarantee that the information is correct and current. He does not, however, guarantee that the data will be error-free or that it will satisfy any certain performance or quality standards. Any negative repercussions that may arise from using or applying the material in this book are not the responsibility of the author, publisher, or distributor.

In this book, references or mentions of individuals, products, websites, organizations, or other names are for informational purposes only and do not imply endorsement or affiliation with the author. The author has no control over the nature, content, and availability of referenced or mentioned entities. Any reliance on such information is at the reader's own risk.

The inclusion of any references does not necessarily imply a recommendation or endorse the views expressed within them. The author or publisher shall not be liable for any loss or damage arising out of or in connection with, the use of this book.

By reading and using the information in this book, you agree to the terms of this disclaimer. If you do not agree with these terms, please refrain from using this book.

INTRODUCTION:

Understanding Esophagitis and the Importance of a Specialized Diet

Esophagitis is the term for the inflammation of the esophagus, the tube that carries food from the mouth to the stomach. Many factors, including infections, allergies, and acid reflux, may be involved in this condition. To properly treat and manage esophagitis, understanding the condition is crucial.

To minimize symptoms and prevent the esophagus from getting worse, a certain diet is necessary.

A diet that reduces acidity and avoids foods that can exacerbate inflammation can be beneficial for those with esophagitis. Usually, this means avoiding alcohol, caffeine, and fatty, spicy, or acidic foods.

A healthy diet can help lessen heartburn, dysphagia, and chest pain. It may also aid in the healing of the esophageal lining.

A tailored diet based on specific requirements and triggers can help people with esophagitis maintain overall digestive health and prevent problems. A tailored diet is therefore essential to the treatment of esophagitis.

CHAPTER ONE

EXPLAINING ACID REFLUX DISEASE

What Is Esophagitis?

The condition referred to as esophagitis is characterized by inflammation or irritation of the esophagus, which is the muscular tube connecting the throat and stomach. It can manifest itself in various ways, ranging from slight discomfort to grave repercussions. Understanding the architecture of the esophagus is crucial to comprehending this condition. The esophagus is crucial to the passage of food and liquids from the mouth to the stomach because it performs a sequence of coordinated muscular contractions known as peristalsis.

Inflammation or irritation of the lining of the esophagus can cause symptoms such as dysphagia, heartburn, regurgitation of food or acidic beverages, and chest pain. These symptoms can significantly lower someone's quality of life by making it difficult for them to eat and causing pain or discomfort when they do.

Esophagitis can be acute or chronic, depending on how long it lasts and how severe the symptoms are. Acute esophagitis often results from brief irritation caused by medicines, infections, or reflux of the stomach acid. Conversely, long-lasting chronic esophagitis has been associated with underlying medical conditions such as gastroesophageal reflux disease (GERD), eosinophilic esophagitis, and Barrett's esophagus.

Understanding the Sources and Symptoms

There are several etiological factors for esophagitis, and each one contributes differently to the disease's progression. One of the main causes is gastric reflux disease (GERD), which is characterized by the reflux of stomach acid backward into the esophagus. This reflux of acidic stomach contents may irritate the lining of the esophagus, causing inflammation and symptoms of esophagitis.

Other common causes of esophagitis include infections, such as those caused by viruses like herpes simplex or fungi like Candida albicans. Individuals with weakened immune systems or those who have undergone specific medical procedures, such as chemotherapy or radiation therapy, are more susceptible to infection.

In addition to infections and gastroesophageal reflux disease (GERD), several medications, particularly those that irritate the stomach lining, can also result in esophagitis. Nonsteroidal anti-inflammatory drugs (NSAIDs), such as aspirin and ibuprofen, have been demonstrated to increase the risk of esophageal irritation and inflammation when taken in high doses or for prolonged periods.

Additionally, individuals with autoimmune illnesses like systemic sclerosis or eosinophilic esophagitis may experience esophageal inflammation due to underlying immunological dysfunction. Due to a heightened immune response, these conditions may eventually lead to inflammation and tissue damage in the esophagus.

It is critical to recognize the signs of esophagitis to receive timely diagnosis and treatment. A typical symptom known as "heartburn" is a burning feeling in the chest that can worsen while you're eating or sleeping. If you have dysphagia, it can also be challenging to swallow solid foods or liquids without feeling uncomfortable.

Other common symptoms of esophagitis include regurgitation of food or sour liquid, which can leave a bitter taste in the mouth, and chest pain, particularly during swallowing or after eating.

Sometimes esophagitis is asymptomatic when it is mild or in its early stages. However, if symptoms worsen or become troublesome, you should consult a physician for further testing to determine the underlying cause and initiate the appropriate course of treatment.

It is easier to diagnose and treat esophagitis when one understands the complex interactions between the various factors that cause the ailment. By treating underlying causes including GERD, infections, or medication-induced irritation, medical practitioners can develop customized treatment plans to lessen symptoms and prevent consequences associated with this illness. To have the greatest outcomes for people with esophagitis, early symptom detection, and prompt treatment are crucial.

CHAPTER TWO

NUTRITIONAL PROTOCOLS FOR THE MANAGEMENT OF ESOPHAGITIS

Understanding the Impact of Food Choices:

Understanding the impact that dietary choices can have on esophagitis is crucial before beginning a diet treatment. Food particles directly contact the sensitive lining of the esophagus in cases of esophagitis, which is described as inflammation of the esophagus. Therefore, dietary choices must be carefully considered. Knowing which meals cause discomfort and inflammation is the first step in comprehending this effect. Common offenders include caffeine, spicy foods, and acidic foods like citrus fruits. These medications have the potential to irritate the stomach lining, which could worsen symptoms and delay healing.

It's critical to understand the necessity of both meal planning and quantity control. The lower esophageal sphincter may be overworked after large, heavy meals, causing stomach acids to reflux back into the esophagus. This highlights the significance of deciding to choose smaller, more frequent meals throughout the day. Being aware of one's tolerance limits is also essential. Some people may feel better if they avoid eating late at night since it allows their bodies more time to process before they fall asleep. A person's ability to make proactive decisions that meet their unique needs and sensitivities is enhanced when they are aware of these intricacies.

Since individual responses to specific foods can vary, novices must adopt an experimental mindset. Keeping a food journal to record meals, symptoms, and perceived triggers can be useful in identifying patterns and developing personalized knowledge about how specific foods impact esophageal health. Based on this process of self-discovery, an effective and long-lasting diet plan for treating esophagitis can be developed.

The Benefits of Personalized Nutrition

When it comes to using food to treat esophagitis, there is no one-size-fits-all approach. Recognizing the individuality of each person's dietary needs, sensitivities, and triggers highlights the importance of a customized eating plan. Those who are new to this route must realize how crucial it is to adjust their diet to suit their circumstances if they want to take control of their health and feel empowered.

Developing a customized diet plan requires speaking with medical specialists, such as gastroenterologists or registered dietitians, as they may provide tailored guidance based on the severity of the illness, previous medical issues, and food preferences. To create a thorough and sustainable diet plan, these experts can perform in-depth assessments and take into consideration factors like food intolerances, allergies, and nutritional deficiencies.

 Armed with professional guidance, novices can begin the actual task of implementing a customized nutrition plan. This means consciously eliminating trigger foods that were identified in the trial phase. In the meantime, options that are easy on the esophagus and aid in healing while lowering inflammation can be provided. Selecting whole grains, lean proteins, and non-acidic fruits, for example, can help create a diet that is both balanced and relaxing.

 Meal planning is a key component in the success of a customized diet plan. It is advised that beginners prepare their meals carefully so that they are satisfying as well as nutrient-dense. This can mean experimenting with culinary techniques, testing out new recipes, and gradually expanding your repertoire of esophagitis-friendly dishes. Having a repertoire of go-to meals eases the process of adhering to the customized diet plan and lessens the likelihood of feeling overwhelmed or limited.

Thus, for those who are new to controlling their illness, comprehending the intricate relationship between dietary choices and esophagitis and realizing the importance of a customized diet plan are crucial first steps. By understanding the impacts of specific foods and tailoring their dietary plan, people can traverse this route with clarity and confidence, ultimately promoting optimal esophageal health and overall well-being.

CHAPTER THREE

LAYING THE FOUNDATION FOR A DIET FOR ESOPHAGITIS

Knowing What Food Triggers Are:

Establishing the foundation of your esophagitis diet is mostly dependent on identifying trigger foods that exacerbate your symptoms. Food triggers for esophagitis, or inflammation of the esophagus, are important to recognize and eliminate from your diet because they often result in flare-ups. For novices, this process could seem intimidating, but with a deliberate approach, it becomes more manageable.

Begin by maintaining a thorough food log. After keeping a journal of everything you consume, record any symptoms or discomfort you experience. This comprehensive log will be a helpful resource in the future for identifying patterns. Look for correlations between specific foods and the onset of esophagitis symptoms.

Common trigger foods include chocolate, coffee, acidic or spicy foods, and fatty or fried foods.

You might want to give an elimination diet a try as a beginner. Start by cutting out potential trigger foods from your diet for a couple of weeks. Reintroduce them one at a time gradually, paying attention to how your body reacts. With the aid of this methodical approach, you may identify the precise causes of the symptoms of esophagitis and adjust your diet accordingly.

Speak with medical specialists or nutritionists who specialize in managing esophagitis. Based on your particular dietary needs and symptoms, they can offer tailored advice and support. Getting expert assistance can expedite the procedure and lessen its intimidating nature for novices.

Keep in mind that each person's body responds differently, so you need to be patient. It takes time to identify trigger foods, and you'll get more accurate results if you stick to a consistent method. Moving forward to the next crucial step in building the basis of your esophagitis diet is possible after you have a better understanding of your triggers.

Accepting Ingredients That Are Esophagitis-Friendly:

Adopting esophagitis-friendly products is a crucial step in building your esophagitis diet foundation, following the identification of trigger foods. These are the foods that promote better digestive health and general well-being since they are less prone to cause esophageal irritation and inflammation. It is necessary to take a realistic and supervised approach when navigating this diet component as a novice.

Choose whole foods that are easy on the esophagus and have not been processed. Your esophagitis-friendly diet should be centered around nutritious grains, lean proteins, and fresh fruits and vegetables. These meals support the upkeep of a healthy digestive system in addition to being nutrient-dense.

Include non-acidic fruits (bananas, melons, and pears) in your diet as they are less likely to cause symptoms of esophagitis. Sweet potatoes, spinach, and carrots are great substitutes since they provide essential nutrients without irritating the skin.

Pick lean protein sources like tofu, skinless chicken, and fish. These solutions are less likely to aggravate symptoms of esophagitis and are easier to digest. To preserve their esophageal-friendly qualities, think about preparing them with gentle cooking techniques like baking, steaming, or grilling.

Give whole grains precedence over processed carbohydrates. Excellent options that lessen the chance of irritation and add to a well-balanced diet are brown rice, quinoa, and oats. Additionally, to reduce the chance of aggravating the symptoms of esophagitis, choose dairy products that are low in fat or fat-free.

Try different herbs and spices that provide flavor without irritating the skin. Due to their anti-inflammatory properties, ginger, turmeric, and fennel can improve the flavor of your food without interfering with your esophagitis-friendly diet.

Choosing substances that are esophagitis-friendly entails doing research and putting your digestive health first. By incorporating these components into your diet, you may lay the groundwork for managing and preventing the symptoms of esophagitis. As a novice, concentrate on introducing these items into your meals gradually so that your body may become used to them and flourish on a diet that supports overall health.

CHAPTER FOUR

PUTTING TOGETHER A SUCCESSFUL KITCHEN

Key Components of a Diet for Esophagitis:

Choosing the right items to include in an esophagitis diet is essential for controlling symptoms and accelerating recovery. Meals that are easy on the esophagus, reducing acidity, and avoiding triggers that exacerbate inflammation should be the main priorities. This is a comprehensive list of the essential components for a kitchen that is esophagitis-friendly:

1. Whole Grains: To start, make sure you eat plenty of whole grains, like oats, brown rice, and quinoa. Because of their high fiber content, these grains make a hearty and filling meal foundation without causing severe reflux. In addition, they cause less esophageal irritation than refined grains do.

Practical Tip: When preparing meals, choose whole-grain pasta or rice alternatives. Additionally, whole-grain bread can be a great addition; just be careful to check for any added sugars that might increase the acidity.

2. Lean Proteins: Opt for lean protein sources such as tofu, skinless chicken, and fish. These choices are less likely to cause acid reflux and are gentler on the digestive system. Avoiding fatty meats is advised because they can aggravate pain and inflammation.

Practical Tip: Rather than frying your protein sources, bake, grill, or simmer them. In addition to reducing added fats, this improves meal digestion.

3. Vegetables: Choose non-acidic vegetables like broccoli, carrots, and leafy greens. These vegetables are not only less likely to cause heartburn, but they are also healthier. Steer clear of citrus fruits, tomatoes, and onions as they have a higher acid content.

Practical Tip: To make veggies easier to digest, steam or sauté them. Try different herbs and spices to enhance flavor without increasing the acidity.

4. Non-Citrus Fruits: Despite the occasional prohibition of citrus fruits, there are plenty of non-acidic fruit options. Plenty of bananas, melons, and apples. These fruits are easy on the esophagus and provide essential vitamins and minerals.

Practical Tip: Blend fruits into smoothies or create fruit salads for a refreshing and healthy snack.

5. Dairy alternatives: If you're sensitive to dairy, think about lactose-free or non-dairy alternatives like almond or oat milk. These alternatives provide a smooth mouthfeel without increasing the chance of acid reflux.

Practical Tip: Use non-dairy substitutes for milk or cream when baking or cooking.

6. Good Fats: Eat foods like avocados, almonds, and olive oil to get heart-healthy fats in your diet.

These fats improve flavor and sate appetite without increasing acidity.

Use olive oil for cooking and when drizzling salads. A handful of unsalted nuts would make a satisfying and healthful snack.

7. Herbs and Spices: To enhance the flavor of your food, use flavor-enhancing, stomach-friendly herbs and spices. Tasteful and non-irritating additives are ginger, mint, and basil.

Practical Advice: Experiment with different herb combinations to find flavors that you enjoy and won't make you sick.

Tips For Grocery Shopping

Shopping for groceries requires careful consideration and decision-making if you have esophagitis. The helpful tips that follow will make sure that your shopping trip is both successful and symptom-free:

1. Make a plan in advance: Before you head to the grocery store, take some time to put your weekly meal plan together. Based on the dishes you want to make, make a shopping list. Ascertain that you have all you require to avoid making snap judgments that may not align with your nutritional needs.

Practical Tip: Keep a running list on a notepad or your phone, adding items as you come across them during the week.

2. Shop the Periphery: The perimeter of the supermarket is typically where you'll find fresh produce, lean meats, and dairy alternatives. Spend much of your shopping time there. This will help you avoid the tempting aisles filled with processed foods that could provoke triggers.

Practical Tip: Look for grains, nuts, and seeds in the bulk section to control portion sizes and reduce packaging waste.

3. Examine Product Labels Carefully: Take the time to carefully study product labels to identify any ingredients or potential triggers that might be harmful to your esophagus. Watch out for hidden sugars, acidic compounds, and preservatives.

Practical Advice: Select products with the fewest ingredients by looking for those that are labeled as low-acid or non-acidic.

4. Choose Whole Foods Rather Than Processed: Whenever possible, choose fresh whole foods over processed ones. Fresh veggies, lean meats, and fruits are not only healthier for you, but they are also less likely to include additives that exacerbate esophagitis symptoms.

Practical Tip: To ensure you always have healthful options available, purchase frozen fruits and vegetables if fresh food isn't available.

5. Amass Esophagitis-Friendly Snacks: Set up a snack cupboard that goes well with your diet for esophagitis. It's a good idea to keep non-citrus fruits, nuts, and low-acid crackers on hand to satisfy cravings without ruining your diet.

Practical Tip: Make snack-sized portions ahead of time to grab on the move to reduce the temptation to choose less healthful options.

6. You might want to consider conducting your grocery shopping online if you have trouble navigating a physical store. It's easier to find esophagitis-friendly items thanks to the opportunity to filter them on many online platforms according to dietary preferences.

Practical Tip: Use subscription services for pantry essentials to make grocery shopping easier and ensure you never run out of supplies.

When grocery shopping, use common sense and pay attention to these directions for essential components so that you may stock your kitchen with foods that will support your esophagitis diet. With careful preparation and wise choices, you'll be well on your way to improving overall digestive health and managing symptoms.

40

CHAPTER FIVE

PLANNING MEALS BY HAND TO ALLEVIATE ESOPHAGITIS

A Weekly Meal Planning Guide:

Creating a weekly eating schedule is crucial to managing esophagitis symptoms and promoting healing. A thoughtfully designed meal plan ensures that you're eating soft, pleasant foods that won't damage your esophagus and help you better control how much food you eat. This comprehensive guide can help even newcomers develop a weekly meal plan that will successfully treat esophagitis.

First, figure out what healthy and relaxing foods go into an esophagitis-friendly diet. Pick easy-to-digest foods like cooked vegetables, whole grains, lean meats, and soft fruits. Recall that to reduce irritation, meals that are greasy, spicy, or acidic should be avoided.

Next, plan your weekly meals, and to keep your diet interesting, be sure to include a range of foods and a good balance of nutrients. The daily objective should be two to three snacks and three main meals. To maintain your energy and aid in recuperation, divide your fats, proteins, and carbohydrates equally.

When planning meals, consider the texture of the food. Select softer foods such as well-cooked vegetables, pureed soups, and tender meats that are easier on the esophagus. Add wholesome grains (such as oats or quinoa) for additional fiber that won't upset the stomach.

Add a range of protein sources, such as fish, tofu, eggs, and lean chicken. These high-protein foods provide essential nutrients and support the healing process. Be mindful of serving quantities to avoid overindulging, which puts additional strain on the esophagus.

Add a variety of fruits and vegetables to ensure a range of vitamins and minerals. Softer foods such as stewed apples, bananas, and melons may be soothing; citrus fruits, on the other hand, maybe overly acidic. To find out which vegetables are most accepted, try a range of them; you may want to stick with steamed or pureed varieties.

Consider your cooking style. Baking, steaming, and boiling are less taxing on the digestive system than frying or grilling. These methods not only preserve nutrients but also make food more palatable for those with esophagitis.

When you're preparing your meals for the coming week, make a note of anything that aggravates your symptoms. To reduce discomfort and promote recovery, these things must be avoided, even in small doses. Keep a food journal to track your reactions and adjust your diet plan as needed.

Lastly, include some flexibility in your meal plan. Observe the cues from your body and adjust as needed. If you're uncomfortable with a particular dish, try something friendlier instead. Regularly check your diet plan to make sure it is still helping you manage your symptoms of esophagitis.

By following this step-by-step instruction, anyone, even without prior meal planning knowledge, may create a weekly meal plan that is effective and beneficial for relieving esophagitis. Eating with intention and consistency will promote general health and the healing process.

Balancing Nutrients and Taste:

The right combination of flavor and nutrients is essential for an esophagitis patient's diet to be both therapeutic and pleasurable. Adhering to dietary restrictions can be challenging at first, especially for those who are not accustomed to them, but with a purposeful approach, it can become less stressful and more rewarding.

First things first, find out what essential nutrients your body needs to heal as best it can. Proteins, carbohydrates, healthy fats, vitamins, and minerals are vital for the digestive system and overall well-being. Include a balance of these nutrients in your meal planning to promote healing without compromising flavor.

Include lean protein sources including chicken, eggs, tofu, and fish. These solutions provide the building blocks needed for tissue repair along with the ideal amount of fat and acidity. To enhance the flavor without causing skin irritation, try experimenting with different cooking methods such as baking or steaming.

Consuming a variety of carbohydrates is recommended, with a focus on whole grains for fiber and sustained energy. Brown rice, quinoa, and oats are all excellent, stomach-friendly options. Refined or highly processed carbohydrates should be avoided as they may make pain and inflammation worse.

Add foods high in good fats to your diet, like olive oil, avocados, and almonds. These fats provide flavor as well as essential components for overall wellness. Keep an eye on portion sizes to avoid overindulging, as consuming excessive amounts of fat can exacerbate acid reflux.

Focus on colorful fruits and vegetables to ensure a broad range of vitamins and minerals. Because of their flavor and nutritional worth, some fruits, such as melons and berries, can be included; however, other fruits, like berries, may be acidic and should be avoided. If you want to enhance flavor without upsetting your palette, try adding some herbs and mild spices.

Consider the general variety and style of your meals. Create aesthetically pleasing food by blending various hues and textures. This increases meal enjoyment and ensures a greater variety of nutrients. To ensure you are getting adequate nutrients and to prevent boredom, mix and match your meals.

Drink water as often as possible to stay hydrated during the day. Avoid caffeine- and carbonated-containing beverages since they can exacerbate acid reflux. When it comes to relaxing options such as diluted fruit drinks or herbal teas, moderation is key.

Pay attention to serving sizes to prevent overindulging, which puts additional strain on the esophagus. Meals that are smaller and more frequent may be gentler on the stomach and help maintain a regular intake of food.

Finally, don't be afraid to experiment with different flavors and cooking methods. Delicious and satisfying meals can still be made with a variety of foods, even if some may be off-limits. For ideas on creative dishes that meet your dietary limitations, look for cookbooks and websites that are esophagitis-friendly.

You may balance flavor and nutrients in your esophagitis-friendly diet to create meals that are both delightful and beneficial. Experiment with different meal combinations, cooking techniques, and seasonings to find options that improve your health without compromising taste.

CHAPTER SIX

RECIPES FOR FOODS SUITABLE FOR ESOPHAGITIS PATIENTS

Moderate Methods of Cooking:

The first step in navigating the world of meals appropriate for people with esophagitis is to understand mild cooking techniques. These techniques are crucial for preparing nutrient-dense, delicious, and easily digestible foods. Among the variety of gentle cooking techniques, steaming stands out for its ability to preserve nutrients and make digestion easier.

Steaming is an easy way to start cooking for someone who has esophagitis if you're a beginner. Using steam to cook food makes it moist and tender without using a lot of oil or salt. To start, select a variety of crisp, soft vegetables, such as zucchini, carrots, and spinach. Cut them into little pieces and place them to steam over hot water in a steamer basket. Cover the saucepan and let the steam work its magic for a short while to preserve the texture and nutrition of the vegetables.

In addition to steaming, poaching is a gentle cooking technique suitable for anyone following an esophagitis diet. This method involves simmering food in a liquid (typically water or broth) at a low temperature. Even novice poachers can become skilled if they stick to delicate items like fish or chicken breasts. To ensure that the protein absorbs the flavors without becoming overly hot, pour it into the simmering liquid and cook it slowly. The result is a dish that is easy to digest and moist, making it a perfect fit for the dietary guidelines for esophagitis.

Furthermore, slow cooking demonstrates its value as an asset for novice cooks. Slow cooking ensures that nutrients break down gradually throughout cooking, which results in more tender and more digested meals. Less-experienced cooks should try combining lean proteins, soft vegetables, and minimal to no spice in their esophagitis-friendly stews, soups, or casseroles.

Since flavors are added gradually while cooking, neither fragile digestive systems nor taste receptors are offended.

For people who are new to the esophagitis diet, using moderate cooking techniques gives up a world of culinary possibilities without losing health. Kids quickly gain proficiency in steaming, poaching, and slow cooking, which transforms the kitchen into a cozy and delicious meal preparation area.

Wonderful and Comforting Recipes:

The cornerstone of the esophagitis diet is developing recipes that are tasty without being overly harsh on the digestive system, ensuring that meals are both easy on the stomach and pleasing to the taste buds. Beginners embarking on this culinary journey may initially find the restrictions on particular items intimidating, but with creativity and thoughtful planning, they may elevate their meals to new heights of flavor.

Using herbs and mild spices in your cooking is an essential strategy for delicious but esophagitis-friendly meals. Fresh herbs, such as basil, chives, and parsley, can add a burst of flavor without overpowering the taste. Novice cooks can experiment with adding these herbs to salads, steamed vegetables, or poached proteins to enhance flavor while adhering to dietary restrictions.

Citrus fruits, in addition to herbs, provide another approach to enhance flavor without making esophagitis symptoms worse. Inexperienced cooks can try sprinkling a small amount of lemon or lime juice over their dish to give it a refreshing acidity that tickles the taste buds without making them sick. Citrus and a range of proteins, like chicken and fish, combine nicely to balance digestibility and flavor.

Choosing lean, delicate cuts of protein is essential to creating satisfying, non-aggravating meals. Beginners can opt for fish, turkey, or chicken breast, all of which can be cooked gently using steaming or poaching methods. These proteins enable novice cooks to create a wide range of delicious dishes that nonetheless follow the exacting requirements of the esophagitis diet.

Furthermore, experimenting with diverse flavor sources, such as broth-based sauces, might enhance the eating experience for individuals who are new to the esophagitis diet. Even novice cooks can enhance the flavor and complexity of their food by starting with a simple broth (prepared from chicken or vegetables) and using it as the base for sauces. When these sauces are applied to slow-cooked stews, poached proteins, or steamed vegetables, they provide a calming flavor layer that doesn't bother.

Fruit that is naturally sweet and soft is a terrific option for sweets that are safe for persons with esophagitis. A lovely way to end a supper without upsetting anyone is to serve baked apples or poached pears that have been lightly seasoned with cinnamon. By adopting these tasty yet non-aggravating recipes, beginners on the esophagitis diet can go on a culinary adventure that not only improves their health but also satisfies their cravings for tasty and cozy meals.

Main Simple and Delicious Recipes Using Ingredients That Are Esophagitis-Friendly:

Cooking using items that are good for esophagitis doesn't have to be hard. Recipes can be prepared using easily digested elements that lessen irritation, yet still taste good. Let's take a look at a few recipes that can help novices prepare foods that are easy on the neck and reflux.

1. Roast the butternut squash until it is tender before making Creamy Butternut Squash Soup. Blend it with a tiny bit of ginger, veggie broth, and salt. The result is a smooth, calming soup that is easy to make and won't exacerbate esophagitis symptoms. Heat it for a hearty meal.

2. For baked chicken with herbs, marinate chicken breasts in garlic, thyme, rosemary, and olive oil. Bake the chicken for perfectly done and tender results. Tasty but simple, this dish provides

a good amount of lean protein without relying on spicy or acidic components that can irritate the esophagus.

3. Quinoa salad with avocado and cucumber: Combine cooked quinoa with diced avocado, cucumber, and a light vinaigrette made with lemon juice and olive oil. This mild salad is a high-nutrient, esophagitis-friendly option that's enjoyable to prepare and eat.

4. Banana-Berry Smoothie: Blend ripe bananas, berries, and almond milk to make a nutrient-rich, relaxing smoothie. This recipe ensures a smooth texture without using any dairy products or potentially uncomfortable acidic fruits. It's a delicious and satisfying option for a snack.

These recipes show you how simple it is to make esophagitis-friendly food without sacrificing flavor. By adding these easy meals to their routine, people can enjoy a range of delicious options while also supporting their esophageal health. Remember to consider personal tolerances and make appropriate adjustments.

5. Ginger-Turmeric Carrot Soup: Sauté chopped carrots, ginger, and turmeric in a pot with a small amount of olive oil until the carrots are soft. Add the vegetarian broth and boil until smooth, then blend. This soup is warming and comforting, but because it contains anti-inflammatory spices like ginger and turmeric, it's also kind on the esophagus.

6. Before baking, cod fillets are marinated in a solution of lemon juice, dill, and salt. After baking, the fish should flake easily. This meal is a great substitute for people who have esophagitis because it is light and flaky and has a fair amount of protein without the acidity of other marinades.

7. To load bell peppers with spinach and quinoa, prepare the quinoa and mix it with chopped tomatoes, sautéed spinach, and a little garlic. Cut the bell peppers in half, pack the insides, and bake until the insides are tender. This recipe provides a high-nutrient, plant-based, easily digestible option with a variety of flavors and textures.

8. Eggs and Spinach: Whisk the eggs together and gently scramble them with the sautéed spinach in a nonstick pan. Season with a pinch of salt and pepper. This easy-to-prepare, high-protein breakfast option won't cause reflux reflux disease. Spinach and eggs combine well to provide all the nutrients you want without compromising flavor.

9. Banana Almond Butter Smoothie Bowl: Blend ripe bananas with almond butter and almond milk to create a smooth and creamy basis for a delicious smoothie bowl. For some texture, top with sliced strawberries, chia seeds, and granola. This aesthetically pleasing, nutrient-dense breakfast or snack substitute is also gentle on the esophagus and satisfies cravings for a nutritious treat.

CHAPTER SEVEN

DELICIOUS BREAKFASTS FOR A GENTLE START

Nutrient-Rich Breakfast Ideas:

1. Smoothie Bowls with Healing Ingredients:

Start your day with a nutrient-packed smoothie bowl that is not only delicious but also gentle on your esophagus. Choose ingredients that promote healing, such as ripe bananas, soothing yogurt, and anti-inflammatory berries.

Consider adding a tablespoon of honey for sweetness and its potential healing properties. To make it even more nutritious, toss in some chia seeds for added fiber and omega-3 fatty acids. The smooth texture of the blended ingredients ensures an easy swallow, making it an ideal choice for those on an esophagitis diet.

Step-by-Step Guide:

1.   Gather your ingredients: ripe bananas, yogurt, berries, honey, and chia seeds.

2.   Blend the bananas, yogurt, and berries until smooth.

3.   Add honey to taste and blend again.

4.   Pour the smoothie into a bowl.

5.   Sprinkle chia seeds on top for added nutrition.

6.   Enjoy your nutrient-rich and soothing smoothie bowl.

2. Oatmeal with Healing Additions:

A warm bowl of oatmeal can be a comforting and nutritious breakfast option for individuals with esophagitis. Opt for steel-cut oats and cook them with almond milk for a smooth consistency. Incorporate sliced bananas for natural sweetness and a soft texture. To enhance the healing properties, consider adding a touch of ground flaxseed, which is rich in omega-3 fatty acids and may contribute to reducing inflammation.

Keep the flavors mild by adding a sprinkle of cinnamon, a spice that is gentle on the digestive system.

Step-by-Step Guide:

1.   Choose steel-cut oats and almond milk for a gentle base.

2.   Cook the oats according to the package instructions.

3.   Slice bananas and add them to the cooking oats.

4.   Stir in ground flaxseed for added nutrition.

5.   Sprinkle a touch of cinnamon for flavor.

6.   Allow the oatmeal to cool slightly before enjoying this nourishing breakfast.

3. Soft Scrambled Eggs with Vegetables:

Scrambled eggs can be an excellent source of protein for breakfast, and they can be prepared in a way that is gentle on the esophagus. Opt for soft scrambled eggs by cooking them slowly over low heat.

Incorporate finely chopped vegetables like spinach, zucchini, or bell peppers for added nutrients. Cooking the vegetables until they are soft ensures an easy swallow. Consider seasoning with a pinch of salt and herbs for flavor without irritating.

Step-by-Step Guide:

1.   Crack eggs into a bowl and whisk them gently.

2.   Heat a non-stick pan over low heat.

3.   Pour the eggs into the pan and stir slowly as they cook.

4.   Add finely chopped vegetables and continue stirring.

5.   Cook until the eggs are soft and the vegetables are tender.

6.   Season with a pinch of salt and herbs for added flavor.

7.   Enjoy your soft scrambled eggs with gentle vegetables.

4. Banana Pancakes with Almond Flour:

For a delicious and esophagus-friendly pancake option, try making banana pancakes with almond flour. Almond flour provides a soft texture, and ripe bananas contribute natural sweetness. The absence of traditional flour makes this a gluten-free option that may be more tolerable for those with esophagitis. Top the pancakes with a dollop of Greek yogurt for additional creaminess and a dose of probiotics, which can be beneficial for digestive health.

Step-by-Step Guide:

1.   Mash ripe bananas in a bowl.

2.   Add almond flour to the mashed bananas and mix well.

3.   Heat a non-stick pan over medium heat.

4.   Spoon the batter onto the pan to form small pancakes.

5.   Cook until the edges are golden brown, then flip and cook the other side.

6.   Serve with a dollop of Greek yogurt for added creaminess.

7.   Enjoy your gluten-free banana pancakes for a satisfying breakfast.

Quick and Easy Morning Options:

1. Greek Yogurt Parfait with Soft Granola:

A quick and easy breakfast option that is gentle on the esophagus is a Greek yogurt parfait with soft granola. Choose a plain, low-fat Greek yogurt for its soothing properties. Layer it with a soft granola that is easy to chew and swallow. Add sliced strawberries or kiwi for a touch of sweetness and additional vitamins. This parfait is not only quick to assemble but also provides a good balance of protein and fiber for a satisfying start to your day.

Step-by-Step Guide:

1.   Spoon Greek yogurt into a bowl or glass.

2.   Layer with a soft granola of your choice.

3.   Add sliced strawberries or kiwi for sweetness.

4.   Repeat the layers until the bowl or glass is filled.

5.   Allow it to sit for a minute to soften the granola slightly.

6.   Enjoy your quick and easy Greek yogurt parfait.

2. Avocado Toast with Soft Whole Grain Bread:

Avocado toast is a simple and nutritious breakfast that can be adapted for an esophagitis-friendly diet. Choose soft whole-grain bread that is easy to chew. Mash ripe avocado and spread it onto the bread. Sprinkle with a pinch of salt and pepper for flavor without irritating. To add extra nutrients, consider topping it with finely chopped tomatoes or a drizzle of olive oil. The creamy texture of avocado makes this a satisfying and quick morning option.

Step-by-Step Guide:

1.   Choose soft whole-grain bread for easy chewing.

2.   Toast the bread to your desired level of crispiness.

3.   Mash ripe avocado and spread it onto the toasted bread.

4.   Sprinkle with a pinch of salt and pepper for flavor.

5.   Top with finely chopped tomatoes or a drizzle of olive oil.

6.   Enjoy your quick and nutritious avocado toast.

3. Chia Seed Pudding with Mashed Berries:

Chia seed pudding is a convenient breakfast option that can be prepared the night before for a quick morning meal. Mix chia seeds with almond milk and let it sit in the refrigerator overnight to thicken. In the morning, top the pudding with mashed berries for added flavor and healing properties.

Chia seeds are rich in fiber, which can be beneficial for digestion, and the soft texture of the pudding makes it easy to swallow.

Step-by-Step Guide:

1.   Mix chia seeds with almond milk in a bowl or jar.

2.   Stir well and refrigerate overnight to thicken.

3.   In the morning, top the pudding with mashed berries.

4.   Stir the berries into the pudding for added flavor.

5.   Enjoy your quick and easy chia seed pudding.

4. Herbal Tea and Non-Acidic Toast with Nut Butter

For a simple yet soothing morning option, consider pairing a cup of non-acidic herbal tea with a slice of whole-grain toast topped with nut butter. Choose a mild herbal tea such as chamomile, ginger, or peppermint, as these options are gentle on the digestive system and can provide a calming start to your day.

Select a whole-grain bread that adheres to your esophagitis diet guidelines, ensuring it is free from acidic additives. Toast the bread to your preferred level of crispiness and spread a layer of nut butter such as almond or sunflower seed butter. Nut butter adds a creamy texture while providing healthy fats and protein to keep you satisfied throughout the morning.

This breakfast option is not only quick to assemble but also a warm and comforting way to begin your day. The combination of herbal tea and non-acidic toast with nut butter offers a balanced mix of hydration, nutrients, and gentle flavors.

5.   Non-Acidic Fruit Smoothie with Oatmeal

Blend a nutritious and easy-to-digest morning option by creating a non-acidic fruit smoothie paired with a side of oatmeal. In a blender, combine non-acidic fruits like bananas, mangoes, and blueberries with a base of almond milk or non-citrus fruit juice. Add a handful of oats to the mixture for added fiber and a subtle thickness.

Blend until smooth and pour the smoothie into a glass. Alongside the smoothie, prepare a bowl of oatmeal using rolled oats cooked with water or a non-acidic milk alternative. Top the oatmeal with sliced non-acidic fruits such as peaches or strawberries for added sweetness and texture.

This combination of a fruit smoothie and oatmeal provides a well-rounded breakfast with a mix of vitamins, minerals, and fiber. It's an excellent option for those seeking a quick and wholesome morning meal while adhering to the esophagitis diet.

6.   Chia Seed Pudding with Berries

Chia seed pudding is a versatile and make-ahead breakfast option that aligns with the esophagitis diet. To prepare this quick morning dish, mix chia seeds with a non-acidic liquid such as almond milk or coconut milk. Add a natural sweetener like honey or agave syrup to taste, keeping in mind your preference for sweetness.

Allow the chia seed mixture to set in the refrigerator for at least a few hours or overnight. As the chia seeds absorb the liquid, they create a pudding-like consistency. Before serving, top the pudding with a generous portion of non-acidic berries such as raspberries, blueberries, or blackberries.

Chia seed pudding with berries not only offers a delightful texture but also provides a nutritious and fiber-rich breakfast. The make-ahead nature of this option makes it convenient for busy mornings, ensuring you have a satisfying and esophagitis-friendly breakfast ready to enjoy.

7.   Rice Cake with Avocado and Poached Egg

Create a simple and savory morning option by assembling a rice cake topped with avocado and a poached egg. Choose rice cakes that are free from acidic additives, and lightly toast them for added crispiness.

Spread a layer of mashed avocado on the rice cake, providing a creamy and nutrient-dense base. In a separate pot, poach an egg until the whites are set but the yolk remains slightly runny. Carefully place the poached egg on top of the avocado-covered rice cake.

This breakfast option offers a combination of complex carbohydrates, healthy fats, and protein. It's a quick and satisfying choice for those seeking a savory start to the day while adhering to the esophagitis diet.

8.   Non-Acidic Fruit Salad with Cottage Cheese

Craft a refreshing and protein-packed morning option by preparing a non-acidic fruit salad with cottage cheese. Choose a variety of non-acidic fruits such as melons, kiwi, and grapes, and chop them into bite-sized pieces.

In a bowl, combine the mixed fruits with a generous scoop of cottage cheese. Cottage cheese is a rich source of protein and has a mild flavor that complements the sweetness of the fruits without triggering acid reflux.

This fruit salad with cottage cheese provides a balance of vitamins, minerals, and protein to kickstart your day. It's a light and energizing breakfast option that can be assembled quickly for those hectic mornings.

CHAPTER EIGHT

SATISFYING LUNCHES WITHOUT THE BURN
Lunch Recipes for Esophagitis Relief

Portable and Office-Friendly Options

Ginger Dressed Grilled Chicken Salad:

For anybody following an esophagitis diet, the Grilled Chicken Salad with Ginger Dressing makes a delightful lunch option. This lunch combines lean protein with esophageal-friendly, relaxing foods. To begin, you will need skinless, boneless chicken breasts. Soak them in a mixture of ingredients that are just slightly acidic, such as olive oil, ginger, and a small amount of honey for sweetness. Let the chicken sit in the seasonings for a minimum of thirty minutes.

When it's time to cook, make sure the chicken is cooked through but not overly dry by grilling it until its internal temperature reaches a safe level.

While the chicken roasts, prepare a bed of mixed greens, such as spinach or butter lettuce. These greens are kinder to the stomach and won't exacerbate esophagitis symptoms. Once the chicken is done, slice it thinly and place it onto the leaves.

The ginger dressing is made with grated ginger, a small amount of olive oil, a little honey, and a dash of apple cider vinegar. Use a whisk to fully combine these ingredients. Drizzle the grilled chicken and leaves with the dressing, giving everything a gentle shake to coat evenly. Ginger in the dressing has anti-inflammatory properties that may help relieve esophagitis in addition to adding taste. This delicious and well-balanced grilled chicken salad is a healthy and satisfying lunch option for those who have esophagitis.

Quinoa and stir-fried vegetables:

Quinoa and Vegetable Stir-Fry is another easy lunch option that's perfect for the workplace. Because quinoa is a flexible grain that is easy on the stomach, it's a great choice for persons with esophagitis.

To start, thoroughly rinse the quinoa to remove any bitterness. To improve the flavor, use vegetable broth for water in the recipe as directed on the package.

Meanwhile, prep an array of colorful vegetables, such as bell peppers, broccoli, carrots, and zucchini. These vegetables have a low acidity level and are rich in vital elements. To make them easier to eat, chop them into small pieces. In a pan, heat a small amount of olive oil and sauté the vegetables until they are tender but still somewhat crunchy.

Once the quinoa and vegetables have cooked, combine them in a large bowl. Add some fresh herbs, like parsley or cilantro, for flavor. To add flavor to the dish, make a simple soy ginger sauce using grated ginger, low-sodium soy sauce, and a small amount of honey. After adding the sauce to the quinoa and vegetables, toss everything together gently.

A satisfying, nutrient-dense, and stomach-friendly dish is the Quinoa and Vegetable Stir-Fry. Because it's easy to pack and reheat, it's a wonderful alternative for folks with busy schedules or for taking a lunch break at the office.

Turkey wraps with avocado:

An excellent option for a lunch that is both office-friendly and portable is the Turkey and Avocado Wrap. This recipe combines the highly digestible lean turkey with the creamy texture of avocado. To begin with, choose a whole-grain or low-acid wrap to lessen the chance of exacerbating esophagitis symptoms. Lay the wrapper flat and spread a thin coating of avocado mash on one side.

After that, place thin slices of turkey over the avocado. Turkey is a lean protein source that is less likely to irritate than higher-fat meats. Add some crisp, fresh lettuce leaves for extra texture and a pleasant touch. If you would like, you can add thinly sliced cucumber for an extra crunch.

Consider using a drizzle of olive oil or a small amount of low-fat mayonnaise to enhance the flavor rather than using acidic condiments. To make sure the parts remain securely within, fold the wrap with extreme caution.

This turkey and avocado wrap is a terrific option for those with esophagitis who want a quick and delicious lunch on the go because it's simple to prepare, pack, and enjoy.

Sweet Potato and Lentil Soup:

The Sweet Potato and Lentil Soup is a satisfying and filling option for lunch that is suitable for people with esophagitis. Sweet potatoes are less prone to irritate and have a softer texture than lentils, which are excellent sources of protein and fiber. First, peel and dice the sweet potatoes, and then thoroughly rinse the lentils.

Put the garlic and onions in a big pot and cook them in a little olive oil until they become translucent. After adding the lentils and sweet potatoes to the pot, pour in the low-sodium vegetable broth. To give the soup anti-inflammatory properties, add a tiny bit of turmeric along with moderate spices like coriander and cumin. Cook until the sweet potatoes and lentils are tender.

Once the soup is heated through, use an immersion blender to purée it until it's smooth. This step ensures that there won't be any discomfort when swallowing the soup. Season to taste and add a sprinkling of fresh herbs, such as chives or parsley, if needed.

The Sweet Potato and Lentil Soup is a nourishing and mild lunch option for people with esophagitis, as it is warm and calming for the digestive system. This soup is a simple and soothing dinner that can be prepared in advance and reheated.

Salmon pieces paired with asparagus:

For a low-acid and omega-3-rich vegetable option for lunch, try the Salmon and Asparagus Parcels. This recipe is a delicious and gentle way to enjoy the healthy fat content of salmon. After gathering the asparagus stalks and fresh salmon fillets, prepare the oven to a moderate temperature.

Place each salmon fillet on a large enough piece of parchment paper so that the fish and vegetables are enclosed. Add a little pepper, salt, and dill to the fish to give it some additional flavor. Arrange some asparagus spears close to the fish, and create a neat and secure package, fold the edges of the parchment paper bundles, and seal them.

Once the salmon is cooked through and the asparagus is tender, bake the packages in the oven. The salmon is kept juicy by the parchment paper's ability to retain moisture. This cooking method minimizes the need for additional fats or acidic ingredients, making it beneficial for those with esophagitis.

Serve the salmon and asparagus parcels with a side of quinoa or a little amount of well-cooked brown rice for a well-balanced and satisfying meal. The omega-3 fatty acids in salmon contribute to a balanced diet and may alleviate symptoms of esophagitis by lowering inflammation.

CHAPTER NINE

RELAXING DINNERS TO END YOUR DAY
Dinnertime Comfort Food Recipes

Salmon with a herb coating and steamed vegetables served over quinoa

Grilled salmon is a fantastic choice for a soothing dinner that complies with the esophagitis diet. Salmon is an excellent source of protein that doesn't cause acid reflux and is high in omega-3 fatty acids. To begin this recipe, marinate the salmon in a mixture of lemon juice, olive oil, and fresh herbs like parsley and dill. Let the salmon absorb these flavors for at least 30 minutes.

While the salmon marinates, prepare the herbed quinoa. Cook the quinoa according to the package's instructions after giving it a good rinse to remove any bitterness. To add taste, add a little salt, a drizzle of olive oil, and chopped herbs like basil and thyme. Quinoa provides the fish with a delicious flavor boost and a nice texture.

As the primary ingredients combine, steam an array of vibrantly colored vegetables. Pick easy-to-digest vegetables like zucchini, carrots, and spinach. Give them a brief steam to retain their nutrients and make them gentler in the digestive system.

Once everything is ready, grill the marinated salmon until it's perfectly flaky. Place the prepared vegetables on one side and the grilled salmon on top of the quinoa that has been flavored with herbs. In addition to being tasty and aesthetically beautiful, this dish is also easy on the esophagus and a delightful treat for the sensations of taste.

Roast turkey and sweet potatoes with a creamy mash

For those with esophagitis, mashed sweet potatoes are a terrific addition to your dinner repertoire because they offer a soothing alternative to typical mashed potatoes. Before starting to make the dish, peel and chop the sweet potatoes into uniform-sized pieces.

Once they become tender to the fork, boil them and blend them using a small amount of almond milk, olive oil, and cinnamon. These elements not only enhance the flavor but also contribute to a creamy texture without the need for any acidic ingredients.

Place the mashed sweet potatoes next to the cooked turkey. Turkey is a lean protein, thus it's usually okay for those with esophagitis. To improve the flavor, marinate the turkey in a mixture of garlic, rosemary, and a tiny bit of low-acid broth. Roast it until it's well done and beautifully browned.

Serve the creamy mashed sweet potatoes beside the succulent roasted turkey. This satisfying and satisfying dinner fits the esophagitis diet rules thanks to the delicious turkey and the creamy sweet potatoes.

Feel free to serve a side of steaming green beans, or any other non-acidic vegetable, to round off the meal.

Stir-fried vegetables over brown rice with tofu

For a light and easily digestible plant-based lunch, try a stir-fried vegetable dish with brown rice and tofu. This recipe follows the esophagitis diet and provides a balanced blend of protein, fiber, and other nutrients.

Press the tofu to remove excess moisture before chopping it into bite-sized cubes. A low-acid stir-fry sauce made with ginger, tamari, or low-sodium soy sauce, and a tiny bit of sesame oil can be used to marinate tofu. Let the tofu absorb the flavors for a minimum of fifteen minutes.

While the tofu is marinating, prepare the stir-fried vegetables. Choose easy-to-digest vegetables like bell peppers, broccoli, and snap peas. Cut them into pieces of the same size to ensure consistent cooking. In a nonstick skillet or wok, stir-fry the tofu and vegetables over medium-high heat until they are crisp-tender.

Cook brown rice according to package directions in the meantime. Brown rice, being a complete grain, adds a nutritious touch to the meal without being too heavy.

Combine the cooked brown rice with the stir-fried tofu and vegetables for a colorful and satisfying supper. For those searching for a filling, esophagitis-friendly dinner, this visually stunning and delicious stir-fried vegetable dish with tofu and brown rice is a terrific option.

Strategies to Avoid Heartburn at Night

Meal timing and portion control

Avoiding heartburn at night requires careful meal preparation and portion control. To give your body enough time to digest before falling asleep, try to eat dinner two or three hours before going to bed.

Eating smaller, more frequent meals during the day rather than large, heavy dinners is another strategy to reduce the likelihood of acid reflux at night.

To make this strategy work, set up a routine that includes your bedtime and plan your meals ahead of time. If dinner and bedtime are later than usual, consider having a little evening snack. Make sure it contains foods that are good for esophagitis, such as a banana or a small dish of non-acidic yogurt.

Elevated Sleep Position

The way you sleep at night greatly affects how heartburn feels during the day. You can prevent the reflux of stomach acid into your esophagus by using wedge pillows or sturdy blocks to elevate the head of your bed. This gradient helps gravity retain stomach contents where they belong, which reduces the likelihood of reflux during the night.

When using this technique, be sure to gradually raise the elevation; you want to aim for an angle that is between thirty and forty-five degrees. To find the most effective and cozy elevation for your unique needs, experiment with different wedge heights and cushion sizes.

It could take some getting used to this new sleeping position, so be patient and adjust as necessary to get the most comfort.

Modifications to Lifestyle

Along with dietary concerns, there are a few lifestyle modifications that might help avoid heartburn at night. Avoid lying down immediately after eating as this can aggravate acid reflux. Instead, engage in easy workouts like taking a stroll or some time spent sitting up straight.

Since stress exacerbates heartburn symptoms, learning stress-reduction tactics may be helpful. Incorporate relaxation techniques like deep breathing, meditation, or gentle yoga into your nightly routine to promote a calm and contented state before bedtime.

It's also a good idea to wear loose clothing to avoid putting unnecessary strain on the stomach, which can exacerbate acid reflux. Select comfortable bedding that allows for unrestricted movement and lessens the pressure on the abdomen.

Drinking Customs

For overall health, it's critical to drink enough water, but timing and technique of hydration are crucial to prevent heartburn at night. Aim to limit the amount of drinks consumed shortly before bed to lessen the possibility of reflux. Instead, make it a point to drink plenty of water during the day and less in the last few hours before bed.

Chewing down and swallowing air can exacerbate reflux and bloating; therefore, take your time and limit your intake to non-acidic beverages such as water, herbal teas, or diluted fruit juices. By including these water habits into your routine, you can enhance digestive health and lessen the likelihood that experiencing heartburn at night will prevent you from getting enough sleep.

Orientation and Movement After Meals

Proper posture and movement after eating can aid in digestion and reduce the risk of nighttime heartburn. Instead of unwinding or going to sleep after eating, stand or sit up straight for at least thirty minutes. This helps food travel through the digestive tract by allowing gravity to do its work, preventing stomach contents from leaking back into the esophagus.

Consider taking a leisurely walk after dinner to enhance digestion and general wellness. Vigorous physical activity should be avoided for an hour after eating since it can increase intra-abdominal pressure and worsen acid reflux. Finding a balance between modest movement and sustaining an erect posture is crucial for heartburn prevention at night.

CHAPTER TEN

TREATS AND SNACKS THAT AREN'T TEMPTING
Healthy Snack Alternatives:

To preserve overall health and enjoyment when managing esophagitis through diet, selecting appropriate snack selections is essential. It can be challenging to decide what to eat for a snack, but you can take advantage of the chance to nourish your body without putting yourself through unnecessary discomfort. Let's examine a variety of options that fulfill the dietary requirements of those with esophagitis and offer a delightful culinary experience.

1. Fresh Fruits: A dish of fresh fruit makes a quick and healthful snack. Opt for less acidic fruits and vegetables, such as bananas, melons, and pears. These fruits are easy on the esophagus and provide essential vitamins and fiber. To add some curiosity, try cutting them into bite-sized pieces or creating fruit salads. This enhances the snack's visual appeal and makes it more accessible for those who struggle with swallowing.

2. Yogurt Parfaits: Greek yogurt's creamy texture and probiotic benefits make it an excellent base for a healthful snack. Place soft fruits like berries or mangoes atop the granola. The granola not only gives the dish a delightful crunch, but it also soothes the esophagus. Verify that the granola is free of allergens like citrus or too much acidity.

3. Whole Grain Crackers with Hummus: When paired with whole grain crackers, a mildly homemade hummus makes for a satisfying and healthful snack. Select crackers that require the least amount of extra spice and ensure that the hummus is made with components that won't cause you any discomfort. Hummus, which is made with chickpeas, olive oil, and a tiny bit of garlic, is a flavorful but mild option.

4. Smooth nut butter: Almond or cashew butter, for example, is a delicious and nutritious snack. Spread them on bread or whole-grain crackers for a delicious combination. Because of their high content of healthy fats, these nut butter can be an excellent source of energy without irritating. Make choices that are low in added sugar and/or salt.

5. Vegetable Sticks with Avocado Dip: Thinly sliced bell peppers, carrots, and cucumbers make excellent appetizers that dip. To enhance the flavor and smoothness, try serving them with a mild avocado dip. Avocados are not only delicious but also a great source of healthy fats. Crunchy vegetables with a creamy dip are a satisfying snack that fits the esophagitis diet plan.

6. Baked Sweet Potato Fries: Are you in the mood for something savory and crispy? Baked sweet potato fries are a great alternative to conventional fries. Sweet potatoes are less acidic and have a softer feel. Cut them into fries, toss them in a little olive oil, and bake until they are caramelized. To bring out the taste without overloading the palate, use mild herbs as a seasoning.

By incorporating these wholesome snack options into your esophagitis diet, you can put your health first and give it more diversity and satisfaction. To find the combinations that suit your taste preferences and dietary needs the best, try out a few different combinations.

Sweets That Won't Give You the Goosebumps:

You don't have to give up desserts to treat reflux disease. If you carefully select your ingredients and cooking methods, you can enjoy sweet foods without causing discomfort. Let's examine some treats that follow the esophagitis diet guidelines so you may have fun without worrying about your health.

1. Cinnamon-Baked Apples: Baked apples are a filling and delectable dessert option that won't make esophagitis symptoms worse. After slicing and coring, mix the apples in cinnamon and bake until tender. Owing to the natural sweetness of the apples and the warming properties of the cinnamon, this dish appears rich but gentle on the esophagus.

2. Chia Seed Pudding: You can easily customize this healthful and versatile dessert to suit your preferences. Chia seeds should be blended with an acidic liquid, like almond or coconut milk. To add even more sweetness, you can top it with a honey drizzle or fresh berries after letting it cool in the refrigerator. The texture of this pudding is pleasant without being too painful.

3. Banana Oat Cookies: To create these quick and nutritious cookies, mash ripe bananas and mix them with oats. Add a small pinch of cinnamon for flavor. After shaping the batter into biscuits, bake them till golden brown. These cookies are naturally delicious and include no unwanted ingredients. Enjoy them as a guilt-free dessert or snack.

4. Coconut Rice Pudding: Try a soothing coconut rice pudding for a creamy and comforting treat. Once the rice is cooked in coconut milk, add a small amount of honey or maple syrup to make it sweeter. Coconut milk adds richness without the acidity of other dairy products. Garnish with shredded coconut or a pinch of cinnamon for extra taste.

5. Mango Sorbet: Enjoy the tropical sweetness of mango sorbet without worrying about its acidity. Blend some coconut water or non-citrus fruit juice with ripe mangos. The mixture needs to be frozen until it resembles sorbet. This refreshing delight offers a mouthwatering blast of flavor without irritating your esophagus.

6. Ginger-flavored Poached Pears: Poached pears with ginger flavoring are a sophisticated and soothing dessert choice. Ripe pears can be made softer by poaching them in ginger syrup. This recipe is elegant and esophageal-friendly, the sweetness of the pears counterbalanced by the delicate warmth of the ginger.

You can enjoy life's sweetness without endangering your health by including these delicacies in your diet. Dessert time may still be an enjoyable part of your cooking experience if you use some creativity and thorough preparation.

CHAPTER ELEVEN

MANAGING DINING OUT WITH ESOPHAGITIS IN RESTAURANTS

Inventive Ordering Methods:
When eating out with esophagitis, it's critical to use clever ordering strategies to ensure that the meal meets your dietary needs. First and foremost, make use of modern technology by viewing the menu in advance on the restaurant's website. Many restaurants now offer comprehensive online menus so you may peruse options in advance and make informed choices.

When you first get to the restaurant, let the server know if you have any dietary restrictions. Pick a moment when they won't be rushed and carefully lay forth the circumstances. Emphasize the significance of avoiding particular trigger foods, such as fried foods, foods with high acidity or spice, and excessively fattening meals. A pleasant and open exchange of information with the waitress is the foundation of a fantastic dining experience.

Adding personal touches to your order is another effective strategy. Most restaurants are happy to accommodate special requests. For example, find out if an item on the menu can have a trigger ingredient changed or eliminated. Select grilled or steamed food over fried ones to cut down on your consumption, and request sauces and dressings on the side.

Don't forget about serving sizes. Larger portions may cause overindulgence and exacerbate your esophagitis symptoms. Choose smaller portions or ask for a to-go box at the beginning of the meal to portion out an adequate amount to resist the need to overindulge.

If you are unclear about any particular parts or preparation methods, don't be afraid to ask questions. The more information you have about your meal, the better equipped you will be to make choices that will support your esophagitis diet.

Remember that your health comes first and that most wait staff members are kind and willing to assist you if you ask for assistance.

How to Communicate Dietary Needs Effectively:

Understanding how to properly express your dietary needs when dining out can make a big difference in how well you get along with restaurant staff if you have esophagitis. Take the first step by calling the restaurant to inquire if they can accommodate your dietary needs. During this initial information exchange, you can assess the restaurant's willingness to work with you and establish whether it's a decent location to eat.

Introduce yourself to your server as soon as you arrive at the restaurant. Calmly and clearly explain the food restrictions connected to your esophagitis. Be prepared to address any queries the server may have and emphasize which foods and meals should be avoided as trigger foods. By providing this information ahead of time, you lower the chance of order errors and make it easier for the kitchen staff to grasp your standards.

If you feel that there aren't enough options or that the labels aren't clear enough, don't be afraid to ask that any current things be changed. Most restaurants are flexible when it comes to dietary requirements, especially those related to medical conditions. Please request additions, deletions, or alterations to fit your specific needs.

It's also imperative to engage with the waitress in a polite but assertive manner. Stress the gravity of your condition and the need to adhere to your doctor's diet. Speaking with grace and kindness can make a big difference in understanding and teamwork.

If your waiter doesn't seem to know what you should be eating, ask to talk with the chef personally. Being straightforward will allow you to answer any concerns or questions the culinary staff may have and ensure that your message is received appropriately.

Remember that effective communication benefits both sides, so praise the restaurant for their cooperation and acknowledge their efforts to comply with your requests.

You may control your esophagitis and confidently have a good meal in restaurants by employing these techniques.

CHAPTER TWELVE

LIFESTYLE SUGGESTIONS FOR ESOPHAGITIS MANAGEMENT

Methods for Stress Reduction:

Stress management is crucial for esophagitis sufferers since stress exacerbates symptoms and slows down the healing process. Using stress-reduction techniques can significantly impact living a better lifestyle. One helpful method is mindfulness meditation. Finding a quiet place, settling in, and focusing on their breathing are good places for beginners to start. This simple yet powerful method promotes tranquility and helps deflect attention from troubling ideas.

Another helpful tactic is progressive muscle relaxation (PMR). This technique, which involves systematically tensing and relaxing different muscle groups, promotes both mental and physical relaxation. Beginners can incorporate PMR into their daily routine with ease by following the recommended exercises, which are available on the internet or through various apps.

Techniques for deep breathing can be beneficial as well. Beginners can learn diaphragmatic breathing by inhaling deeply through their nose, allowing their abdomen to expand, and then softly expelling through their mouth. Through inducing the relaxation response in the body, this technique reduces stress levels.

If beginners establish a routine, such as dedicating a few minutes each day for relaxation exercises, they could find them simpler to manage. Consistency is key to optimizing the benefits of stress-reduction techniques, building up your tolerance to stress over time, and helping to manage your esophagitis overall.

Engaging in Exercise for a Healthy Digestive System:

Exercise is critical to maintaining digestive health, which is especially important for people with esophagitis. Low-impact workouts are the ideal option for novices to start with to avoid exacerbating symptoms. Walking is a terrific substitute, and beginners can progressively increase the time and pace as they become more accustomed to it.

Yoga is another easy exercise that may be adjusted for newcomers. Certain yoga poses, such as twists and stretches that don't put too much strain on the esophagus, can aid in digestion. Online videos or starting classes can teach one how to safely include yoga in their practice.

Strengthening the core muscles through Pilate's workouts is beneficial for intestinal health. Pilates movements can be started simply by beginners and advanced to more complicated routines. These exercises improve digestion in general and reduce the risk of acid reflux by stabilizing the abs.

Swimming is a low-impact cardiovascular exercise that enhances overall fitness without putting undue strain on the digestive system. Beginners can start with shorter workouts and gradually extend them as their fitness levels develop.

Beginners should consult a healthcare professional or a fitness consultant before starting a new exercise program to ensure that it fits their specific health needs and goals for managing esophagitis. A tailored approach will maximize the benefits of incorporating physical activity into their daily routine.

CHAPTER THIRTEEN

THE PATH TO LONG-TERM ESOPHAGITIS RELIEF

Keeping An Eye On Progress And Adjusting The Diet:

Maintaining a detailed log of your eating habits and symptoms is crucial to achieving long-term treatment for esophagitis. Following up on developments not only provides valuable information about potential trigger meals but also makes it easier to spot trends that help create a personalized and effective diet plan.

Begin by keeping a simple notebook in which you can list all of the meals, snacks, and beverages you consume each day along with any accompanying symptoms, such as reflux, heartburn, or difficulty swallowing. Include the time of consumption and note any external factors, like stress or physical activity. This detailed documentation will serve as a foundation for understanding the relationship between the foods you eat and your esophagitis symptoms.

If you're a novice just starting, consider using technology to streamline processes. Many apps allow users to rapidly log meals and symptoms. Often, these systems include additional features like trend analysis, which makes it easier to spot recurring patterns. Accept these technical tools as a way to improve tracking and the accuracy of your observations.

Look through your notes often to identify any trends or foods that are often linked to negative effects. Keep in mind that various persons may have different triggers for esophagitis, which is why this personalized tracking is crucial. Once trends are established, gradually reduce or eliminate from your diet any foods that have been identified as triggers.

You must modify your diet gradually. Unexpected changes can be daunting and hard to deal with. Instead, go gradually and methodically, allowing your body to acclimate to the changes.

Consider seeing a nutritionist or medical professional to ensure that the dietary adjustments you make will fulfill your nutritional requirements.

Keep a journal that you periodically examine and update as you make dietary modifications. Track any progress or setbacks, and be open to changing your plan of action in response to the outcomes you observe. Ensuring that your diet for esophagitis remains sustainable and effective over time requires this iterative process.

In summary, keeping an eye on your progress and modifying your diet are ongoing, dynamic activities. By using technology, maintaining an extensive notebook, and making little dietary adjustments, even a novice like you can take charge of your esophagitis symptoms and manage them well.

Celebrating Success and Maintaining a Healthier Lifestyle:

Appreciating any progress made in managing esophagitis through dietary changes is an important first step toward a long-term recovery. Not only does acknowledging and reaping the benefits lift one's emotions, but it also underscores how important maintaining a healthy lifestyle is. Here's a beginner's guide to maintaining and enjoying your growth, step by step.

Celebrate your small victories first. Take a moment to celebrate your victories when you see that your symptoms are getting better after making dietary adjustments. Each good improvement—whether it's fewer heartburn episodes or increased comfort during meals—leads to higher esophageal health.

Consider creating milestones to mark significant progress in your management of your esophagitis. These benchmarks could be based on how long you avoid symptoms, how successfully you cut out trigger foods, or how well you stick to your new eating plan. Establishing these benchmarks strengthens your determination to lead a healthy lifestyle and provides you with quantifiable goals.

Consider yourself to grasp the broader impact of your work. Consider how your enhanced nutrition has enhanced your overall well-being and quality of life in addition to your physical health.

You will be greatly motivated to adhere to your esophagitis management goals by this self-examination.

Incorporate a support system into your celebration strategy. Share your triumphs with friends, family, or a support group. It can be uplifting and encouraging to have a network of people who are aware of your path as support. Additionally, it makes group celebrations possible, which fosters a sense of accomplishment and community.

It takes more than food changes to maintain a healthy lifestyle. Accept regular exercise as an extra component of your esophagitis therapy plan. Exercise improves overall health, helps people lose weight, and may reduce acid reflux symptoms. Choose engaging interests to make your workout routine more fun.

Look into stress-reduction techniques to help you better control your esophagitis. Stress can exacerbate symptoms, so including practices like yoga, deep breathing exercises, or meditation in your daily routine may be beneficial.

Partaking in these activities not only improves the health of your esophagus but also improves your whole mental and emotional wellness.

Lastly, think about how long your achievements will be useful. While you celebrate your achievements, remember the principles that have led to these changes. Maintain a diet that is esophagitis-friendly, regular exercise, and stress-reduction techniques as top priorities to ensure that your progress endures.

In conclusion, maintaining a healthy lifestyle and celebrating achievements are critical elements of managing esophagitis. In addition to finding relief, novices with esophagitis can lead fulfilling lives by lowering stress levels, embracing physical activity, establishing goals, celebrating small victories, and building support networks.

MY GRATITUDES

Dear Valued Readers and Supporters,

I hope this message finds you well. I am writing to express my deepest gratitude to both God and each one of you for the overwhelming support and positive response to my book. Your encouragement and enthusiasm have truly touched my heart, and I am immensely thankful for the journey we are on together.

I believe that every success is a result of collaboration and support from various sources. First and foremost, I want to acknowledge the divine guidance and inspiration that led me to create this cookbook. Without the grace of God, this endeavor would not have been possible.

To my cherished readers, your commitment to exploring healthier dietary options for managing your crises has been both inspiring and humbling. Your trust in this book" means the world to me, and I am honored to be part of your journey toward improved health and well-being.

Also, I am reaching out to kindly request your valuable feedback on this book. Your thoughts and insights are crucial in helping me enhance and serve you better, ensuring that it continues to meet your needs effectively. Please take a moment to share your thoughts by rating and writing reviews on platforms where the book is available.

Your reviews not only provide me with invaluable feedback but also play a significant role in assisting others in making informed choices. By sharing your experiences, you contribute to a community that values health and wellness, creating a positive impact on countless lives.

Additionally, I encourage you to share this book with your friends, family and loved ones.

Together, we can extend the reach of this promising resource, offering support and guidance to those who may benefit from it. Having this knowledge and seeking medical advice from your specialist I anticipate a turnaround for us.

Once again, thank you from the depths of my heart for your unwavering support. I am committed to continually improving and serving you better. Let us continue this journey together, promoting health, well-being, and a shared sense of community.

With sincere appreciation,

[Emmy Brooks]

Author, "ESOPHAGITIS DIET COOKBOOK"